Monthly Cycles

Period & PMS Tracker

DEDICATION

This book is dedicated to all the girls or women who want to accurately track their period or menstrual cycle.

Your are my inspiration for producing books and I'm honored to be a part of keeping all your period notes all in one place.

This journal notebook will help you record your periods every month and symptoms.

HOW TO USE THIS BOOK

The purpose of this book is to keep all of your periods, symptoms and mood notes all in one place. It will help keep you organized.

This Period Tracker Journal will allow you to accurately document your monthly flow so you can start to see a pattern with your periods.

Here are examples of the prompts for you to fill in and write about yourself in this book:

1. Month, Year & Undated Calendar - Undated for your convenience.
2. Type Of Flow - Light, Medium, Heavy.
3. Days Since Last Period - Write the day you start & finish.
4. Weight & Temp - Record your weight & temperature.
5. Symptoms - Cramps, Acne, Headaches, Backaches, Bloating, Cravings, Tender Breasts, Nausea, Neck Aches with symptom check boxes.
6. Moods - Track your mood.
7. Things I Did To Feel Better - Write the things that eased your symptoms.
8. Notes - For writing any extra additional or practical information such as pain level, your yearly checkup info, ovulation, or just as a diary to write your feeling & thoughts.

Reminder:

Consult your doctor regularly in matters relating to your health especially with symptoms that may need medical attention and diagnosis.

This tracker is not intended to substitute a doctor's professional medical advice.

Month:

Year:

Sunday	Monday	Tuesday	Wednesday	Thursday	Friday	Saturday

Days Since Last Period:

Count the number of days in between the 1st day of each cycle. Take the average of several cycles and find out how long your cycles are.

Weight:

Temp:

Symptoms:

- ☐ Cramps
- ☐ Acne
- ☐ Headaches
- ☐ Backaches
- ☐ Bloating
- ☐ Cravings
- ☐ Tender Breasts
- ☐ Nausea
- ☐ Neck Aches

Mood:

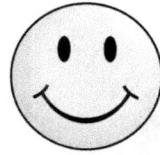

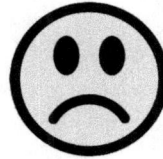

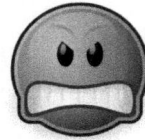

	Things I Did To Feel Better
Day 1	
Day 2	
Day 3	
Day 4	
Day 5	
Day 6	
Day 7	

Notes:

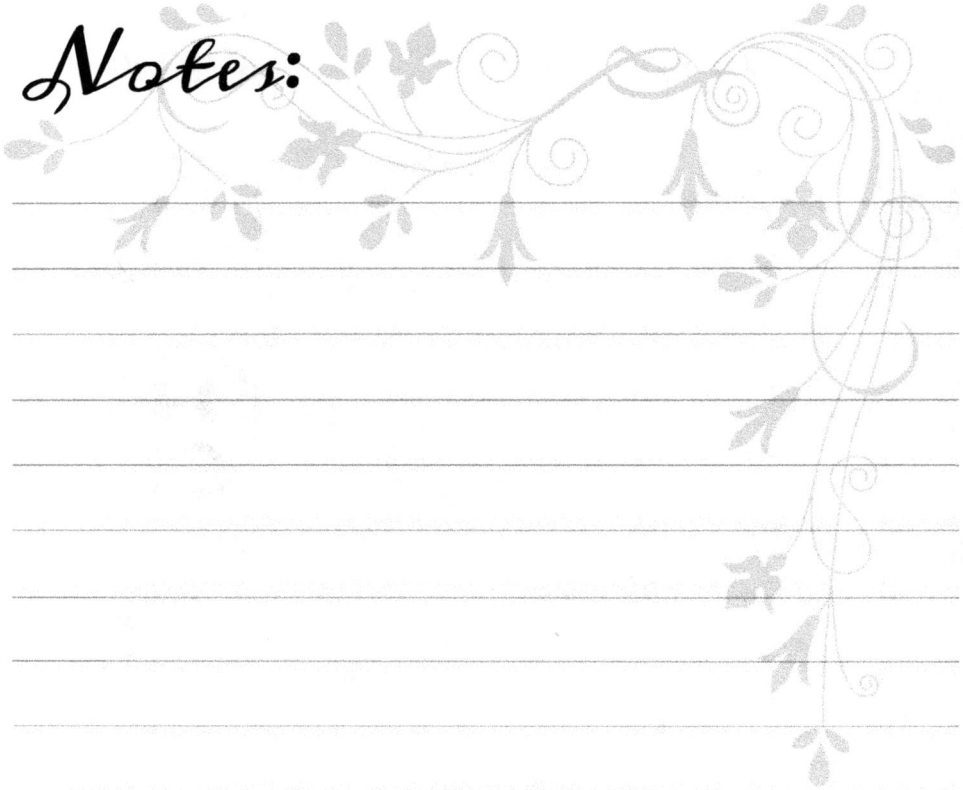

Month:
Year:

Sunday	Monday	Tuesday	Wednesday	Thursday	Friday	Saturday

Days Since Last Period:

Count the number of days in between the 1st day of each cycle. Take the average of several cycles and find out how long your cycles are.

Weight:

Temp:

Symptoms:

- ❏ Cramps
- ❏ Acne
- ❏ Headaches
- ❏ Backaches
- ❏ Bloating
- ❏ Cravings
- ❏ Tender Breasts
- ❏ Nausea
- ❏ Neck Aches

Mood:

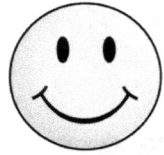

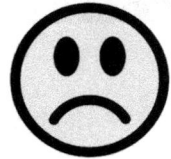

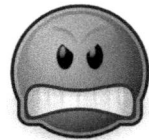

	Things I Did To Feel Better
Day 1	
Day 2	
Day 3	
Day 4	
Day 5	
Day 6	
Day 7	

Notes:

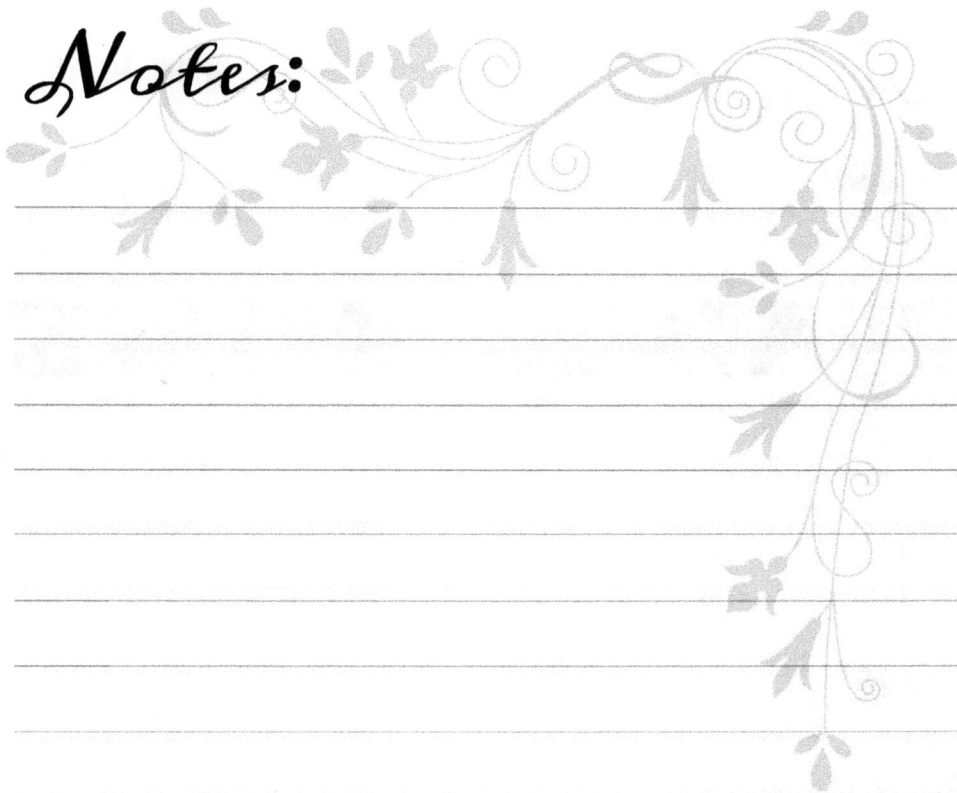

Month:
Year:

Sunday	Monday	Tuesday	Wednesday	Thursday	Friday	Saturday

Days Since Last Period:

Count the number of days in between the 1st day of each cycle. Take the average of several cycles and find out how long your cycles are.

Weight:

Temp:

Symptoms:

- ☐ Cramps
- ☐ Acne
- ☐ Headaches
- ☐ Backaches
- ☐ Bloating
- ☐ Cravings
- ☐ Tender Breasts
- ☐ Nausea
- ☐ Neck Aches

Mood:

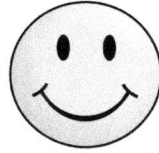

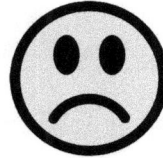

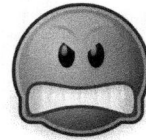

	Things I Did To Feel Better
Day 1	
Day 2	
Day 3	
Day 4	
Day 5	
Day 6	
Day 7	

Notes:

Month:

Year:

Sunday	Monday	Tuesday	Wednesday	Thursday	Friday	Saturday

Days Since Last Period:

Count the number of days in between the 1st day of each cycle. Take the average of several cycles and find out how long your cycles are.

Weight:

Temp:

Symptoms:

- ❏ Cramps
- ❏ Acne
- ❏ Headaches
- ❏ Backaches
- ❏ Bloating
- ❏ Cravings
- ❏ Tender Breasts
- ❏ Nausea
- ❏ Neck Aches

Mood:

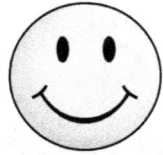

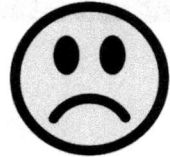

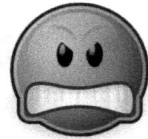

	Things I Did To Feel Better
Day 1	
Day 2	
Day 3	
Day 4	
Day 5	
Day 6	
Day 7	

Notes:

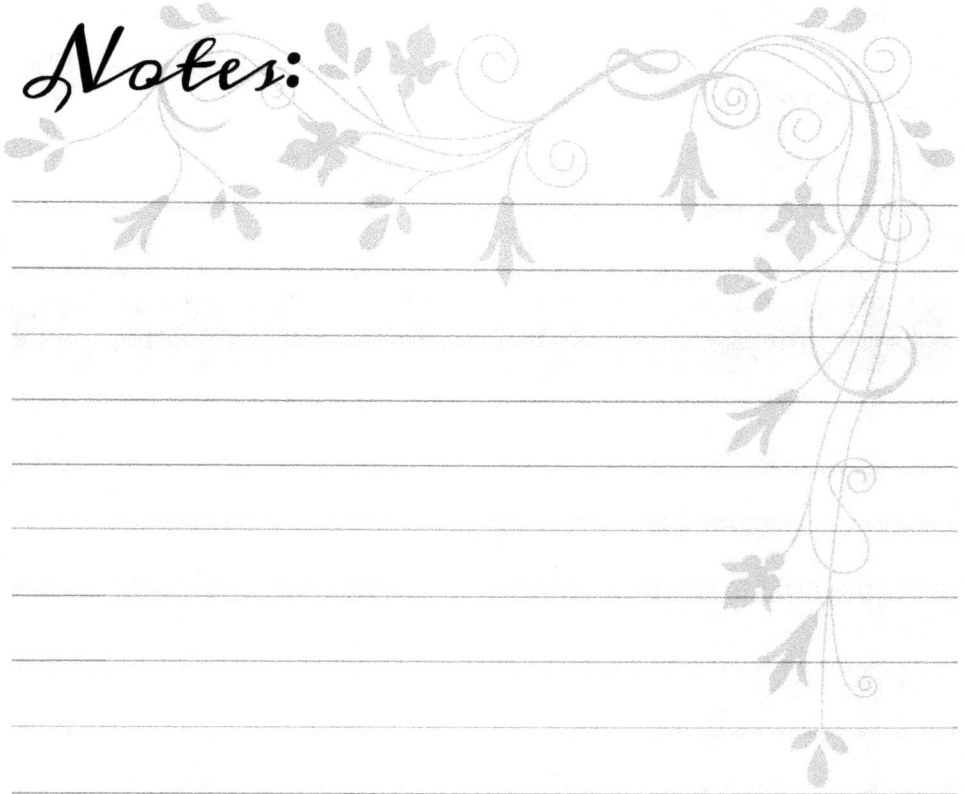

Month:

Year:

Sunday	Monday	Tuesday	Wednesday	Thursday	Friday	Saturday

Days Since Last Period:

Count the number of days in between the 1st day of each cycle. Take the average of several cycles and find out how long your cycles are.

Weight:

Temp:

Symptoms:

- ☐ Cramps
- ☐ Acne
- ☐ Headaches
- ☐ Backaches
- ☐ Bloating
- ☐ Cravings
- ☐ Tender Breasts
- ☐ Nausea
- ☐ Neck Aches

Mood:

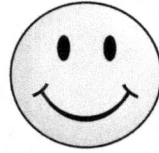

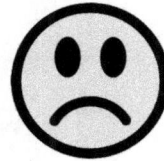

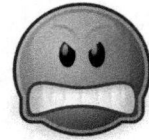

	Things I Did To Feel Better
Day 1	
Day 2	
Day 3	
Day 4	
Day 5	
Day 6	
Day 7	

Notes:

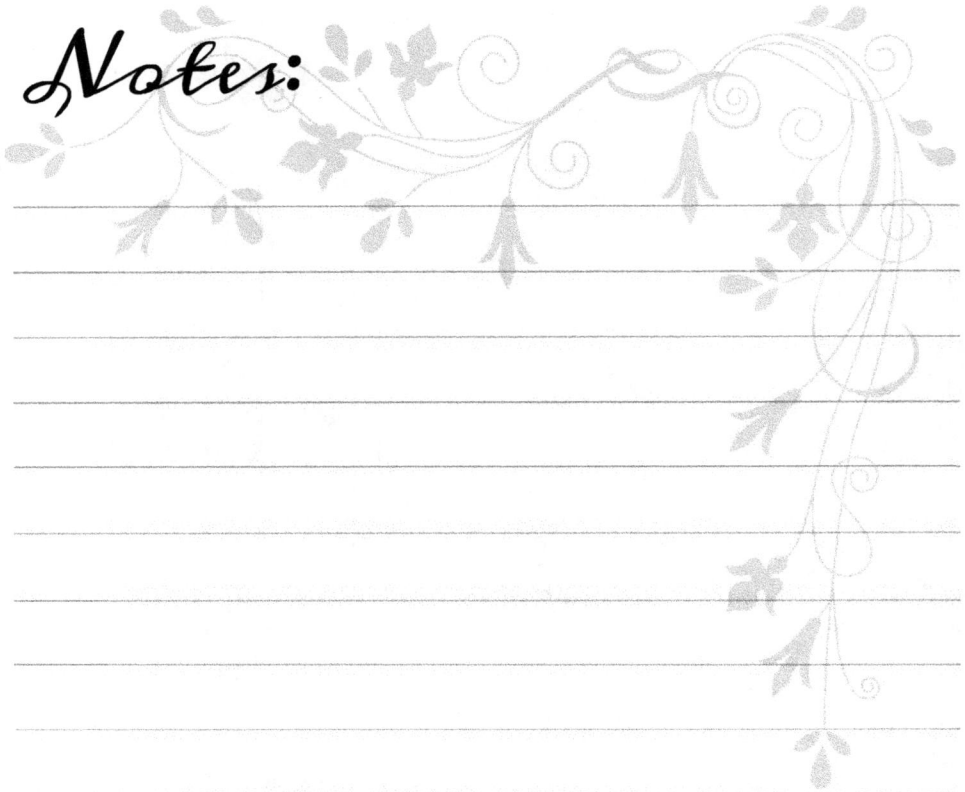

Month:
Year:

Type Of Flow:

L – Light
M – Medium
H – Heavy

Sunday	Monday	Tuesday	Wednesday	Thursday	Friday	Saturday

Days Since Last Period:

Count the number of days in between the 1st day of each cycle. Take the average of several cycles and find out how long your cycles are.

Weight:

Temp:

Symptoms:

- ❏ Cramps
- ❏ Acne
- ❏ Headaches
- ❏ Backaches
- ❏ Bloating
- ❏ Cravings
- ❏ Tender Breasts
- ❏ Nausea
- ❏ Neck Aches

Mood:

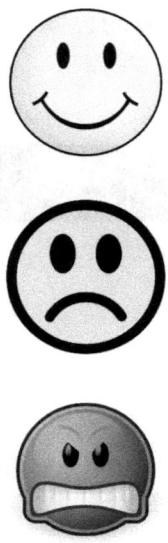

	Things I Did To Feel Better
Day 1	
Day 2	
Day 3	
Day 4	
Day 5	
Day 6	
Day 7	

Notes:

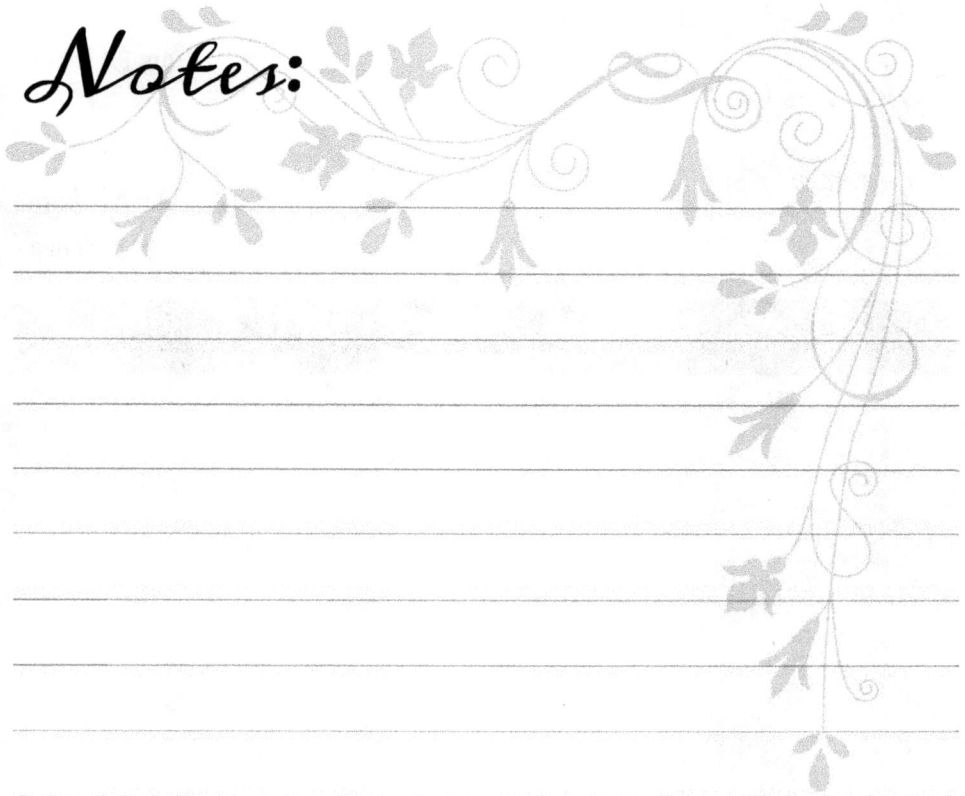

Month:

Year:

Type Of Flow:

L – Light
M – Medium
H – Heavy

Sunday	Monday	Tuesday	Wednesday	Thursday	Friday	Saturday

Days Since Last Period:

Count the number of days in between the 1st day of each cycle. Take the average of several cycles and find out how long your cycles are.

Weight:

Temp:

Symptoms:

- ❑ Cramps
- ❑ Acne
- ❑ Headaches
- ❑ Backaches
- ❑ Bloating
- ❑ Cravings
- ❑ Tender Breasts
- ❑ Nausea
- ❑ Neck Aches

Mood:

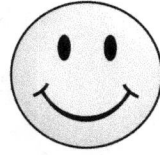

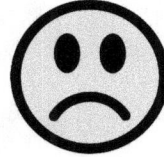

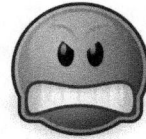

	Things I Did To Feel Better
Day 1	
Day 2	
Day 3	
Day 4	
Day 5	
Day 6	
Day 7	

Notes:

Month:

Year:

Sunday	Monday	Tuesday	Wednesday	Thursday	Friday	Saturday

Days Since Last Period:

Count the number of days in between the 1st day of each cycle. Take the average of several cycles and find out how long your cycles are.

Weight:

Temp:

Symptoms:

- ❏ Cramps
- ❏ Acne
- ❏ Headaches
- ❏ Backaches
- ❏ Bloating
- ❏ Cravings
- ❏ Tender Breasts
- ❏ Nausea
- ❏ Neck Aches

Mood:

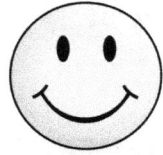

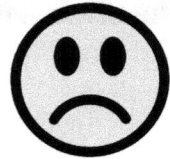

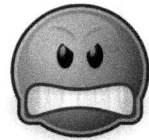

	Things I Did To Feel Better
Day 1	
Day 2	
Day 3	
Day 4	
Day 5	
Day 6	
Day 7	

Notes:

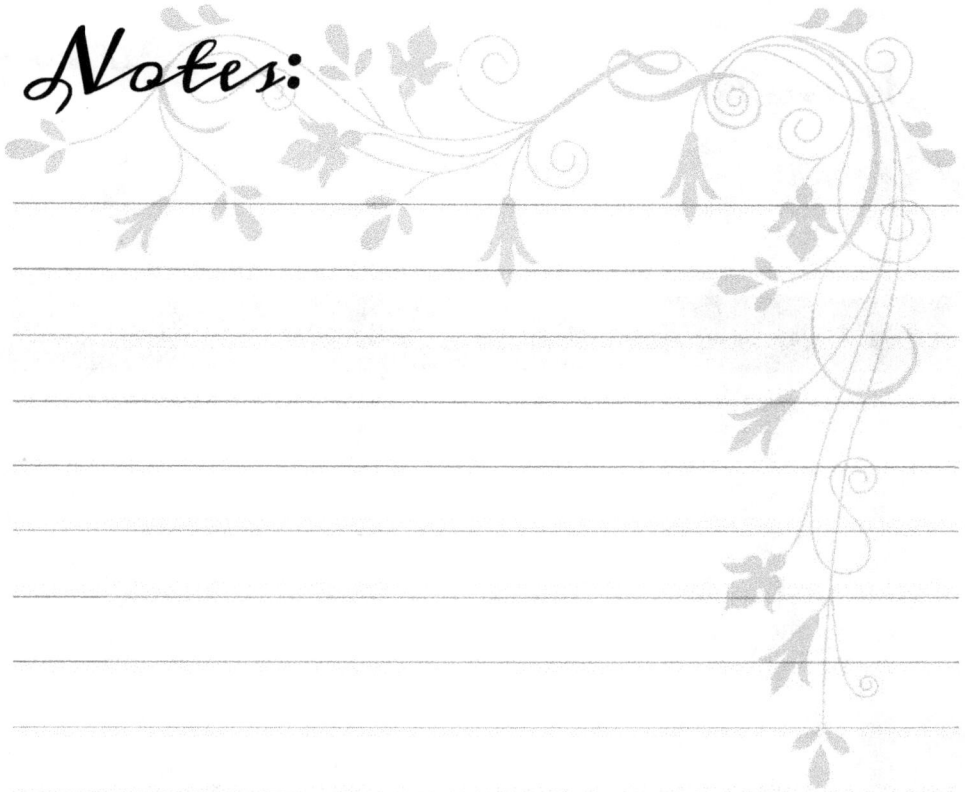

Month:

Year:

Sunday	Monday	Tuesday	Wednesday	Thursday	Friday	Saturday

Days Since Last Period:

Count the number of days in between the 1st day of each cycle. Take the average of several cycles and find out how long your cycles are.

Weight:

Temp:

Symptoms:

- ❏ Cramps
- ❏ Acne
- ❏ Headaches
- ❏ Backaches
- ❏ Bloating
- ❏ Cravings
- ❏ Tender Breasts
- ❏ Nausea
- ❏ Neck Aches

Mood:

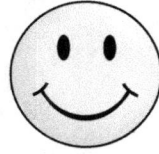

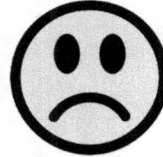

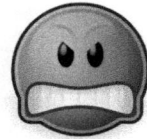

	Things I Did To Feel Better
Day 1	
Day 2	
Day 3	
Day 4	
Day 5	
Day 6	
Day 7	

Notes:

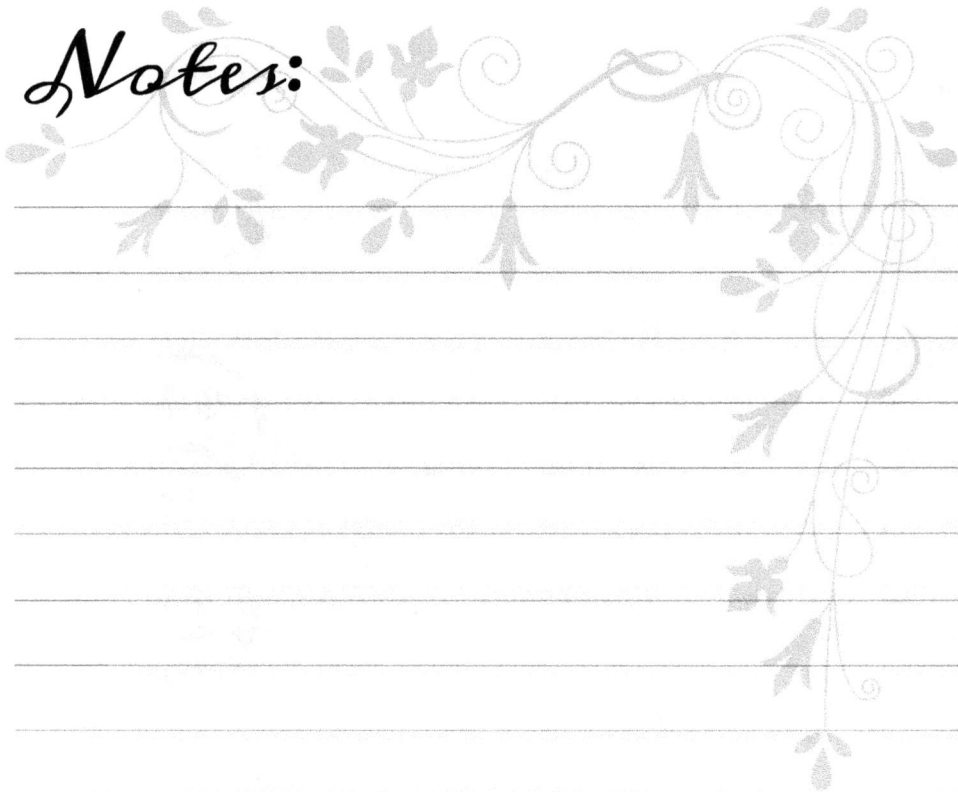

Month:

Year:

Type Of Flow:

L – Light
M – Medium
H – Heavy

Sunday	Monday	Tuesday	Wednesday	Thursday	Friday	Saturday

Days Since Last Period:

Count the number of days in between the 1st day of each cycle. Take the average of several cycles and find out how long your cycles are.

Weight:

Temp:

Symptoms:

- ❏ Cramps
- ❏ Acne
- ❏ Headaches
- ❏ Backaches
- ❏ Bloating
- ❏ Cravings
- ❏ Tender Breasts
- ❏ Nausea
- ❏ Neck Aches

Mood:

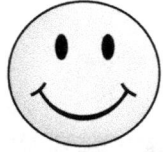

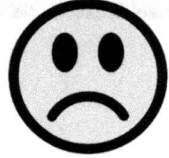

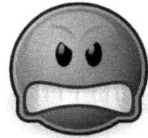

	Things I Did To Feel Better
Day 1	
Day 2	
Day 3	
Day 4	
Day 5	
Day 6	
Day 7	

Notes:

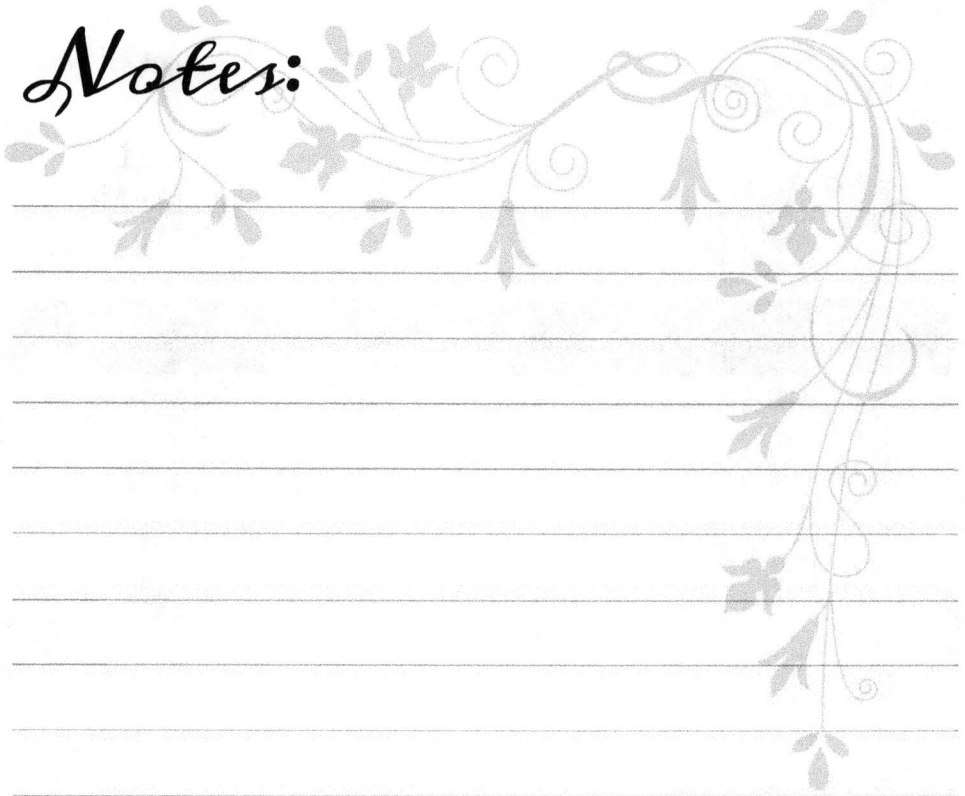

Month:

Year:

Type Of Flow:

L – Light
M – Medium
H – Heavy

Sunday	Monday	Tuesday	Wednesday	Thursday	Friday	Saturday

Days Since Last Period:

Count the number of days in between the 1st day of each cycle. Take the average of several cycles and find out how long your cycles are.

Weight:

Temp:

Symptoms:

- ☐ Cramps
- ☐ Acne
- ☐ Headaches
- ☐ Backaches
- ☐ Bloating
- ☐ Cravings
- ☐ Tender Breasts
- ☐ Nausea
- ☐ Neck Aches

Mood:

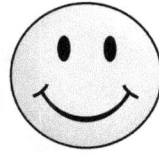

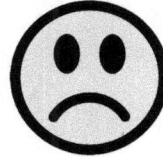

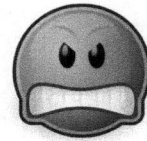

	Things I Did To Feel Better
Day 1	
Day 2	
Day 3	
Day 4	
Day 5	
Day 6	
Day 7	

Notes:

Month:

Year:

Sunday	Monday	Tuesday	Wednesday	Thursday	Friday	Saturday

Days Since Last Period:

Count the number of days in between the 1st day of each cycle. Take the average of several cycles and find out how long your cycles are.

Weight:

Temp:

Symptoms:

- ❏ Cramps
- ❏ Acne
- ❏ Headaches
- ❏ Backaches
- ❏ Bloating
- ❏ Cravings
- ❏ Tender Breasts
- ❏ Nausea
- ❏ Neck Aches

Mood:

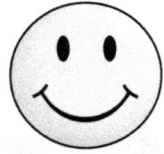

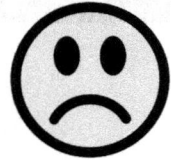

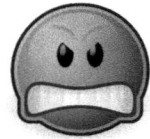

	Things I Did To Feel Better
Day 1	
Day 2	
Day 3	
Day 4	
Day 5	
Day 6	
Day 7	

Notes:

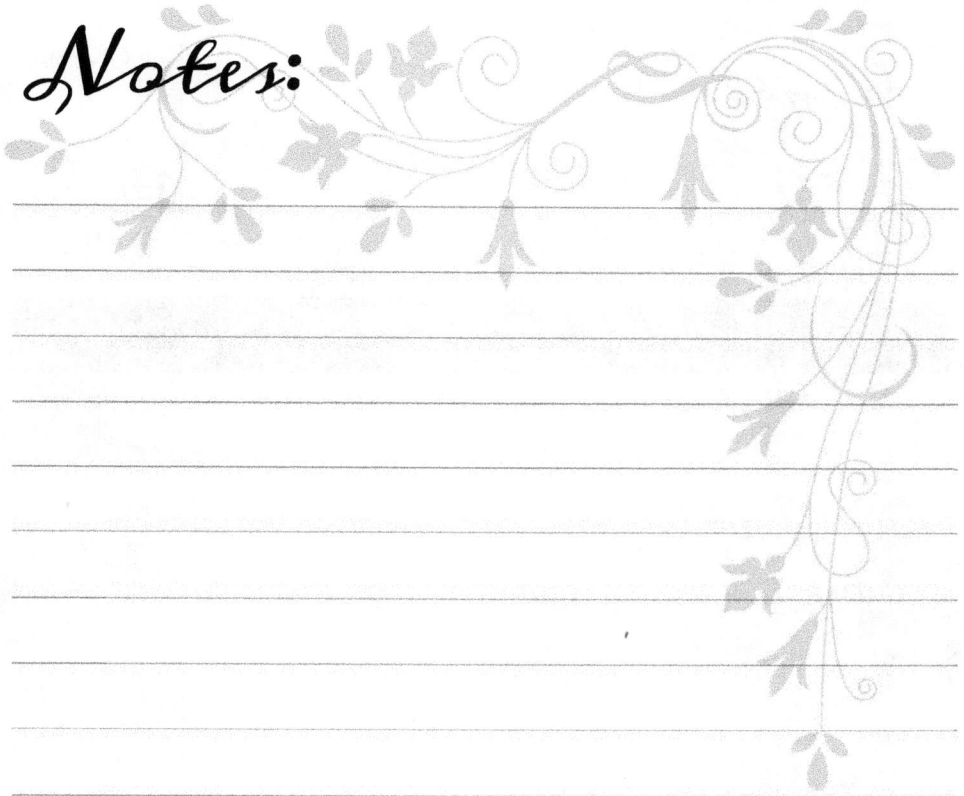

Month:

Year:

Sunday	Monday	Tuesday	Wednesday	Thursday	Friday	Saturday

Days Since Last Period:

Count the number of days in between the 1st day of each cycle. Take the average of several cycles and find out how long your cycles are.

Weight:

Temp:

Symptoms:

- ☐ Cramps
- ☐ Acne
- ☐ Headaches
- ☐ Backaches
- ☐ Bloating
- ☐ Cravings
- ☐ Tender Breasts
- ☐ Nausea
- ☐ Neck Aches

Mood:

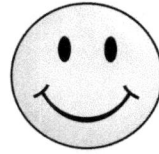

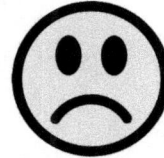

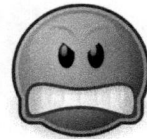

	Things I Did To Feel Better
Day 1	
Day 2	
Day 3	
Day 4	
Day 5	
Day 6	
Day 7	

Notes:

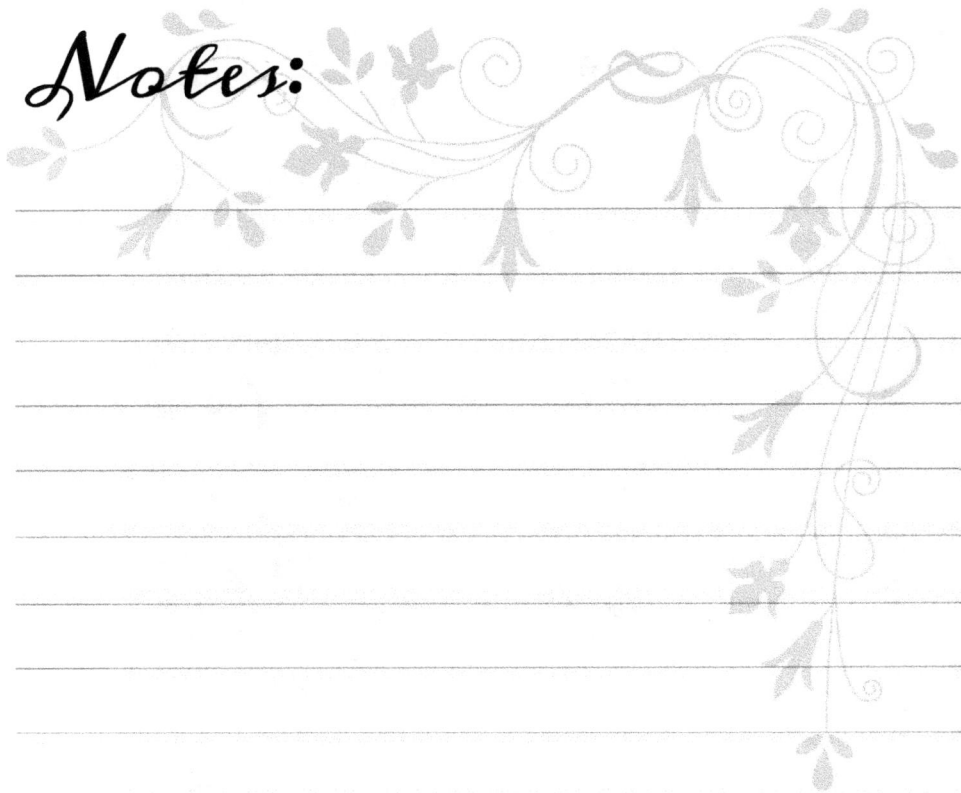

Month:
Year:

Sunday	Monday	Tuesday	Wednesday	Thursday	Friday	Saturday

Days Since Last Period:

Count the number of days in between the 1st day of each cycle. Take the average of several cycles and find out how long your cycles are.

Weight:

Temp:

Symptoms:

- ❏ Cramps
- ❏ Acne
- ❏ Headaches
- ❏ Backaches
- ❏ Bloating
- ❏ Cravings
- ❏ Tender Breasts
- ❏ Nausea
- ❏ Neck Aches

Mood:

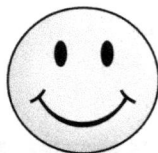

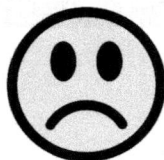

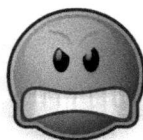

	Things I Did To Feel Better
Day 1	
Day 2	
Day 3	
Day 4	
Day 5	
Day 6	
Day 7	

Notes:

Month:
Year:

Sunday	Monday	Tuesday	Wednesday	Thursday	Friday	Saturday

Days Since Last Period:

Count the number of days in between the 1st day of each cycle. Take the average of several cycles and find out how long your cycles are.

Weight:

Temp:

Symptoms:

- ❏ Cramps
- ❏ Acne
- ❏ Headaches
- ❏ Backaches
- ❏ Bloating
- ❏ Cravings
- ❏ Tender Breasts
- ❏ Nausea
- ❏ Neck Aches

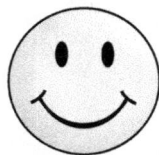

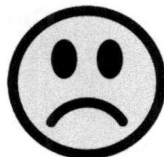

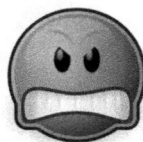

Mood:

	Things I Did To Feel Better
Day 1	
Day 2	
Day 3	
Day 4	
Day 5	
Day 6	
Day 7	

Notes:

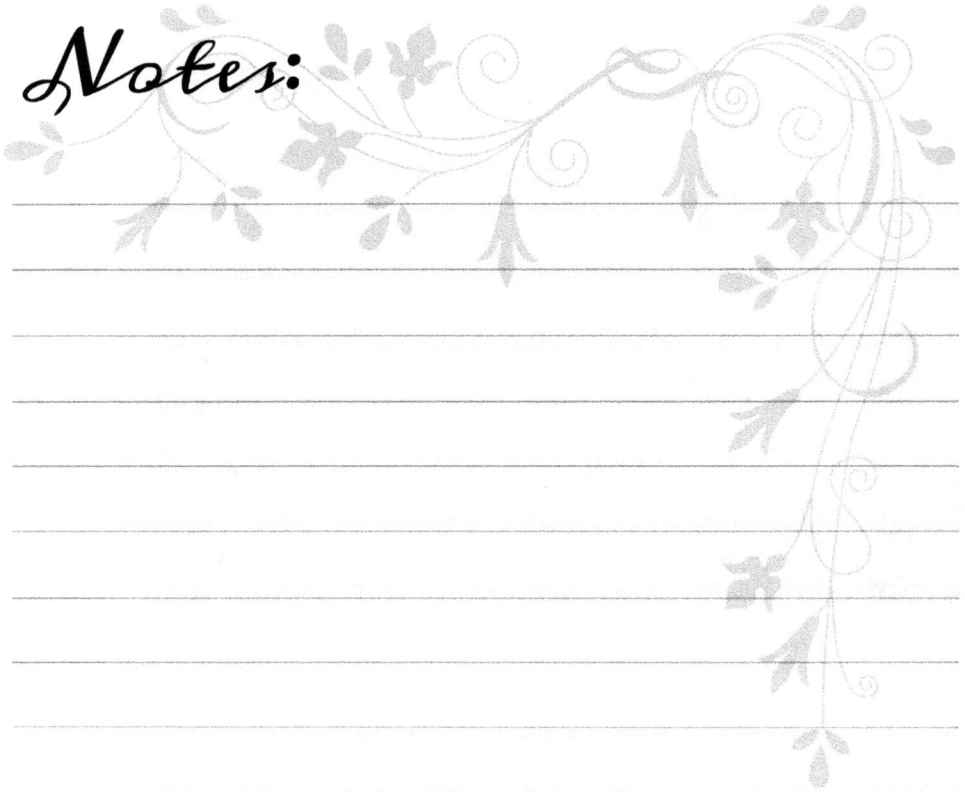

Month:

Year:

Sunday	Monday	Tuesday	Wednesday	Thursday	Friday	Saturday

Days Since Last Period:

Count the number of days in between the 1st day of each cycle. Take the average of several cycles and find out how long your cycles are.

Weight:

Temp:

Symptoms:

- ❏ Cramps
- ❏ Acne
- ❏ Headaches
- ❏ Backaches
- ❏ Bloating
- ❏ Cravings
- ❏ Tender Breasts
- ❏ Nausea
- ❏ Neck Aches

Mood:

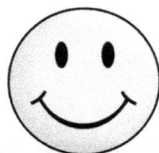

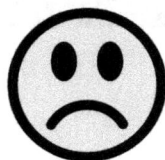

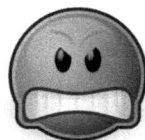

	Things I Did To Feel Better
Day 1	
Day 2	
Day 3	
Day 4	
Day 5	
Day 6	
Day 7	

Notes:

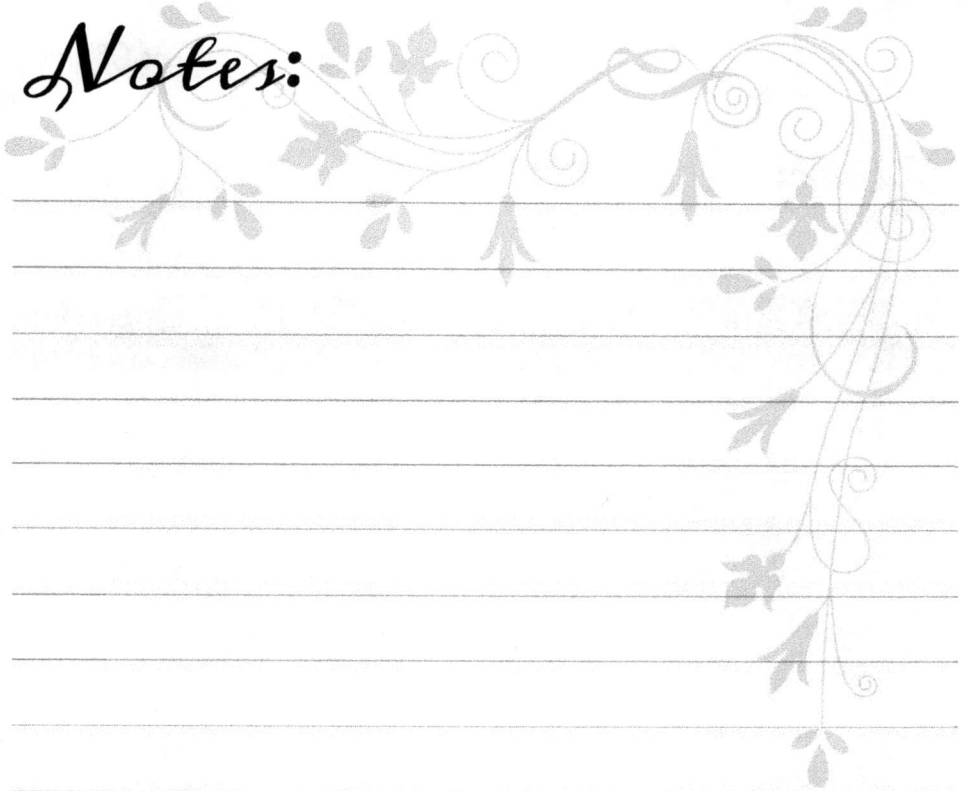

Month:

Year:

Sunday	Monday	Tuesday	Wednesday	Thursday	Friday	Saturday

Days Since Last Period:

Count the number of days in between the 1st day of each cycle. Take the average of several cycles and find out how long your cycles are.

Weight:

Temp:

Symptoms:

- ☐ Cramps
- ☐ Acne
- ☐ Headaches
- ☐ Backaches
- ☐ Bloating
- ☐ Cravings
- ☐ Tender Breasts
- ☐ Nausea
- ☐ Neck Aches

Mood:

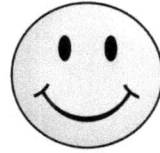

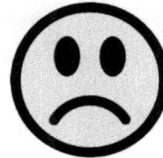

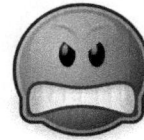

	Things I Did To Feel Better
Day 1	
Day 2	
Day 3	
Day 4	
Day 5	
Day 6	
Day 7	

Notes:

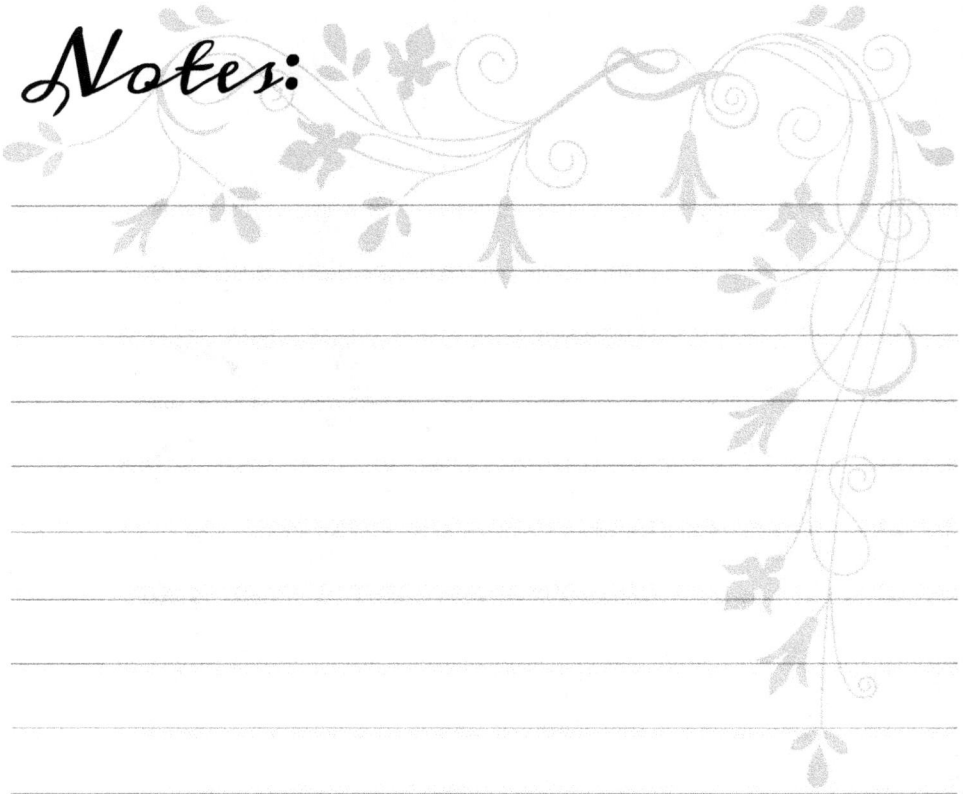

Month:

Year:

Sunday	Monday	Tuesday	Wednesday	Thursday	Friday	Saturday

Days Since Last Period:

Count the number of days in between the 1st day of each cycle. Take the average of several cycles and find out how long your cycles are.

Weight:

Temp:

Symptoms:

- ☐ Cramps
- ☐ Acne
- ☐ Headaches
- ☐ Backaches
- ☐ Bloating
- ☐ Cravings
- ☐ Tender Breasts
- ☐ Nausea
- ☐ Neck Aches

Mood:

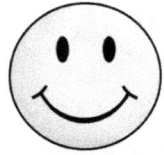

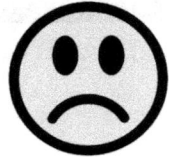

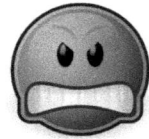

	Things I Did To Feel Better
Day 1	
Day 2	
Day 3	
Day 4	
Day 5	
Day 6	
Day 7	

Notes:

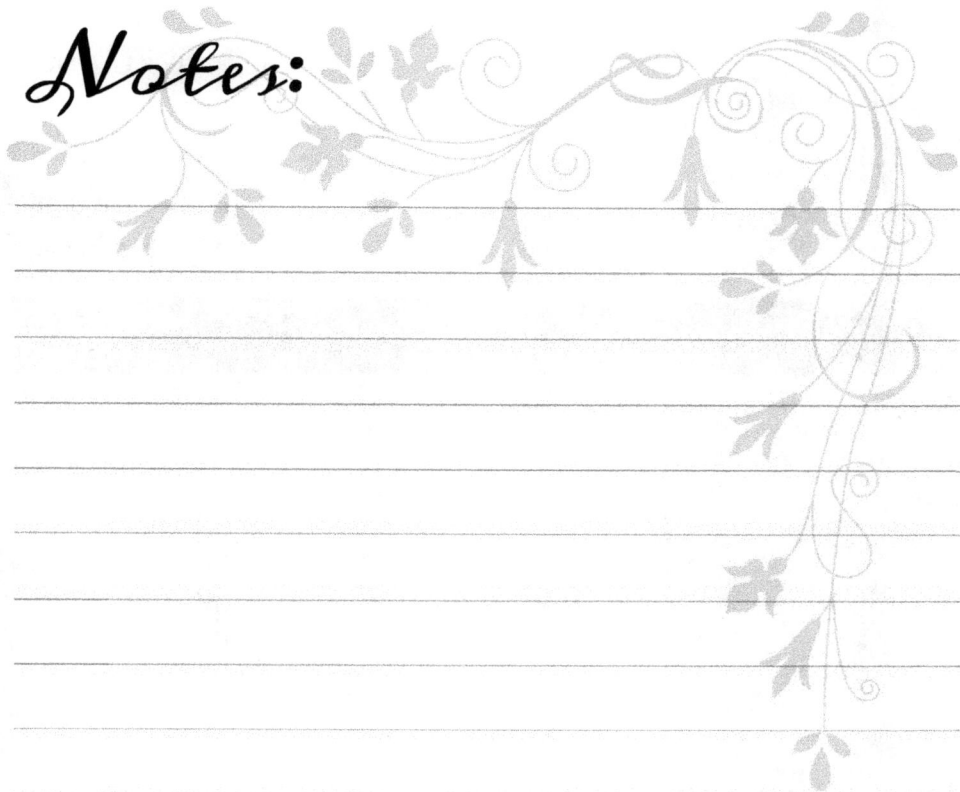

Month:
Year:

Sunday	Monday	Tuesday	Wednesday	Thursday	Friday	Saturday

Days Since Last Period:

Count the number of days in between the 1st day of each cycle. Take the average of several cycles and find out how long your cycles are.

Weight:

Temp:

Symptoms:

- ☐ Cramps
- ☐ Acne
- ☐ Headaches
- ☐ Backaches
- ☐ Bloating
- ☐ Cravings
- ☐ Tender Breasts
- ☐ Nausea
- ☐ Neck Aches

Mood:

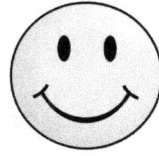

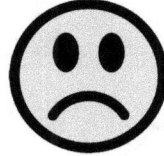

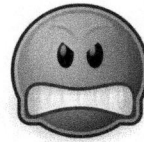

	Things I Did To Feel Better
Day 1	
Day 2	
Day 3	
Day 4	
Day 5	
Day 6	
Day 7	

Notes:

Month:

Year:

Sunday	Monday	Tuesday	Wednesday	Thursday	Friday	Saturday

Days Since Last Period:

Count the number of days in between the 1st day of each cycle. Take the average of several cycles and find out how long your cycles are.

Weight:

Temp:

Symptoms:

- ❏ Cramps
- ❏ Acne
- ❏ Headaches
- ❏ Backaches
- ❏ Bloating
- ❏ Cravings
- ❏ Tender Breasts
- ❏ Nausea
- ❏ Neck Aches

Mood:

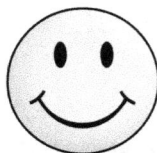

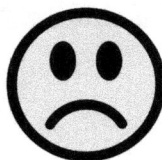

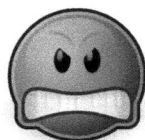

	Things I Did To Feel Better
Day 1	
Day 2	
Day 3	
Day 4	
Day 5	
Day 6	
Day 7	

Notes:

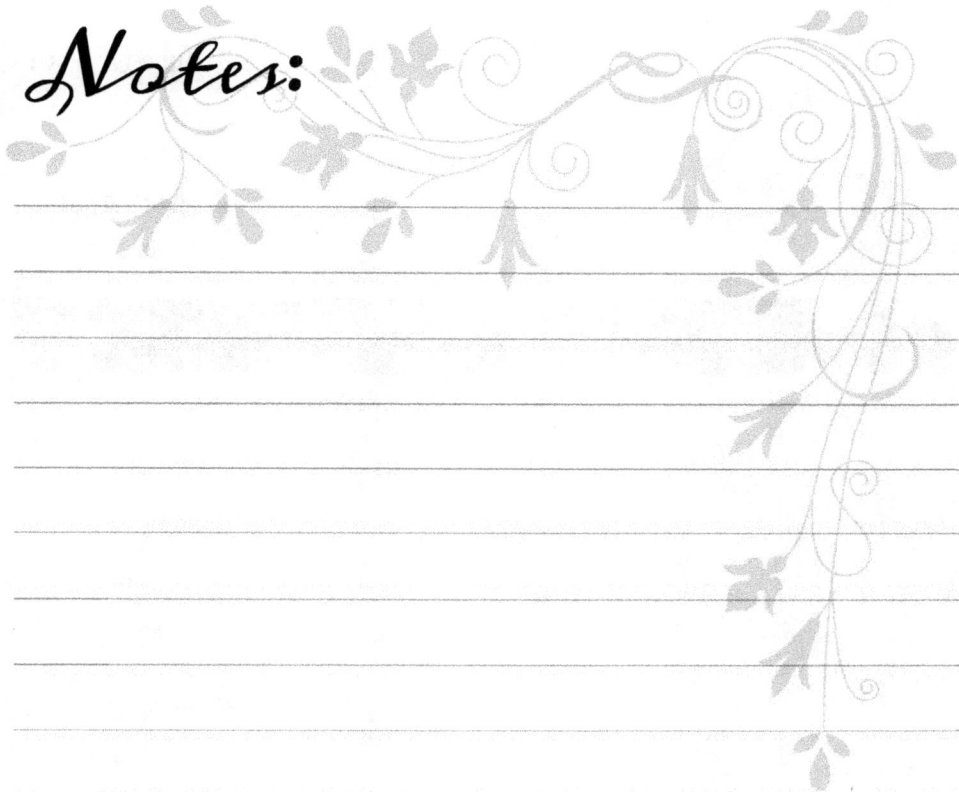

Month:

Year:

Sunday	Monday	Tuesday	Wednesday	Thursday	Friday	Saturday

Days Since Last Period:

Count the number of days in between the 1st day of each cycle. Take the average of several cycles and find out how long your cycles are.

Weight:

Temp:

Symptoms:

- ☐ Cramps
- ☐ Acne
- ☐ Headaches
- ☐ Backaches
- ☐ Bloating
- ☐ Cravings
- ☐ Tender Breasts
- ☐ Nausea
- ☐ Neck Aches

Mood:

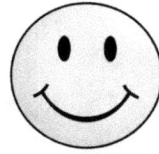

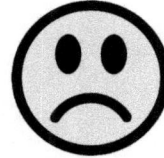

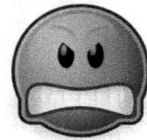

	Things I Did To Feel Better
Day 1	
Day 2	
Day 3	
Day 4	
Day 5	
Day 6	
Day 7	

Notes:

Month:

Year:

Sunday	Monday	Tuesday	Wednesday	Thursday	Friday	Saturday

Days Since Last Period:

Count the number of days in between the 1st day of each cycle. Take the average of several cycles and find out how long your cycles are.

Weight:

Temp:

Symptoms:

- ❏ Cramps
- ❏ Acne
- ❏ Headaches
- ❏ Backaches
- ❏ Bloating
- ❏ Cravings
- ❏ Tender Breasts
- ❏ Nausea
- ❏ Neck Aches

Mood:

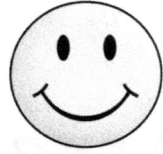

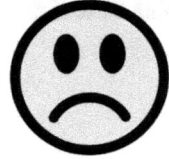

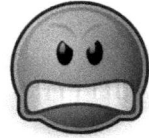

	Things I Did To Feel Better
Day 1	
Day 2	
Day 3	
Day 4	
Day 5	
Day 6	
Day 7	

Notes:
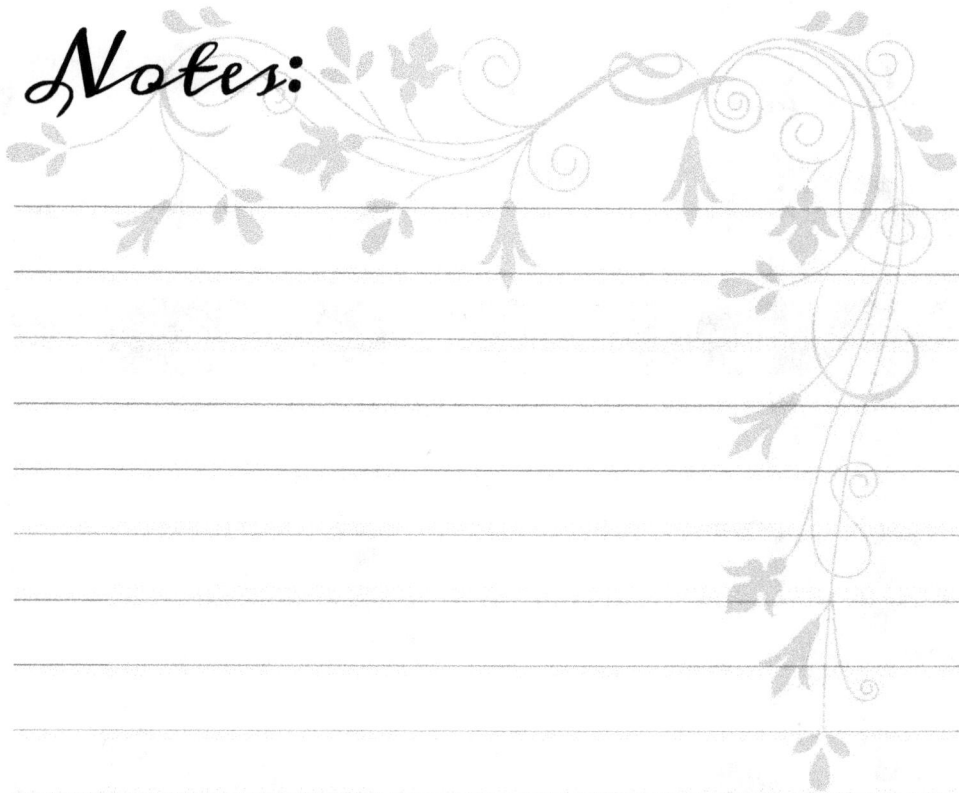

Month:

Year:

Sunday	Monday	Tuesday	Wednesday	Thursday	Friday	Saturday

Days Since Last Period:

Count the number of days in between the 1st day of each cycle. Take the average of several cycles and find out how long your cycles are.

Weight:

Temp:

Symptoms:

- ☐ Cramps
- ☐ Acne
- ☐ Headaches
- ☐ Backaches
- ☐ Bloating
- ☐ Cravings
- ☐ Tender Breasts
- ☐ Nausea
- ☐ Neck Aches

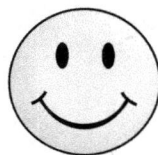

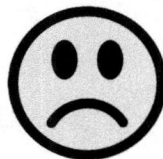

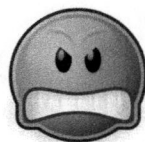

Mood:

	Things I Did To Feel Better
Day 1	
Day 2	
Day 3	
Day 4	
Day 5	
Day 6	
Day 7	

Notes:

Month:
Year:

Sunday	Monday	Tuesday	Wednesday	Thursday	Friday	Saturday

Days Since Last Period:

Count the number of days in between the 1st day of each cycle. Take the average of several cycles and find out how long your cycles are.

Weight:

Temp:

Symptoms:

- ❏ Cramps
- ❏ Acne
- ❏ Headaches
- ❏ Backaches
- ❏ Bloating
- ❏ Cravings
- ❏ Tender Breasts
- ❏ Nausea
- ❏ Neck Aches

Mood:

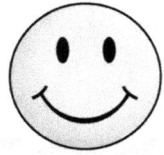

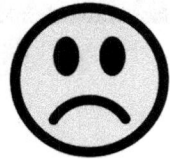

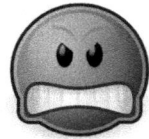

	Things I Did To Feel Better
Day 1	
Day 2	
Day 3	
Day 4	
Day 5	
Day 6	
Day 7	

Notes:

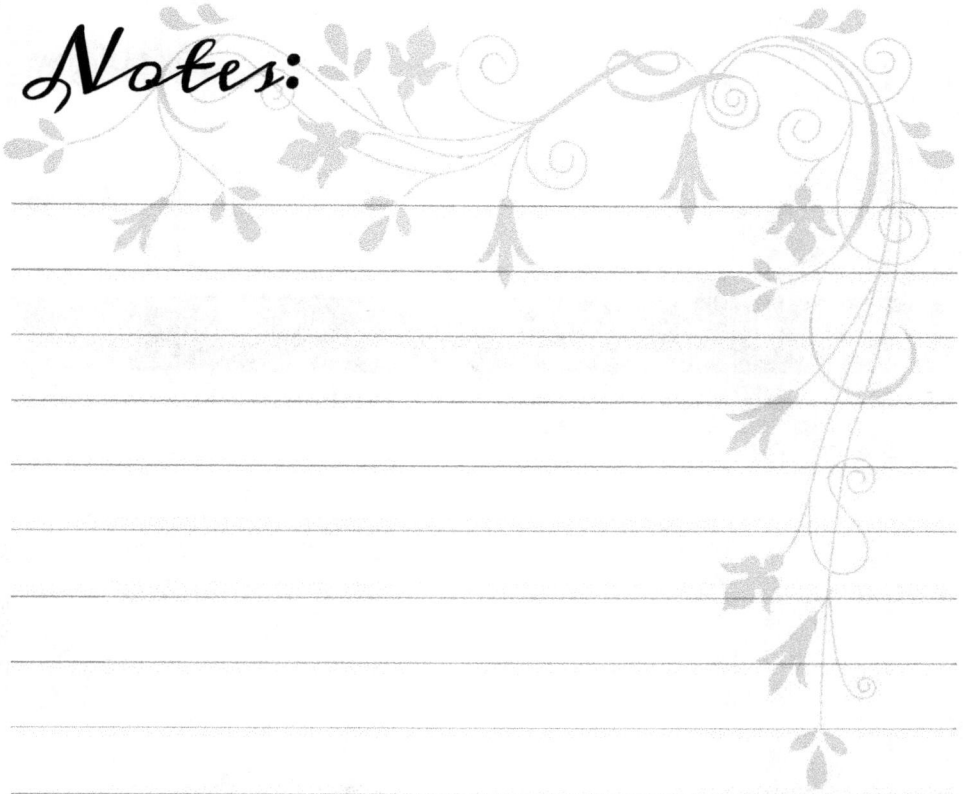

Month:

Year:

Sunday	Monday	Tuesday	Wednesday	Thursday	Friday	Saturday

Days Since Last Period:

Count the number of days in between the 1st day of each cycle. Take the average of several cycles and find out how long your cycles are.

Weight:

Temp:

Symptoms:

- ☐ Cramps
- ☐ Acne
- ☐ Headaches
- ☐ Backaches
- ☐ Bloating
- ☐ Cravings
- ☐ Tender Breasts
- ☐ Nausea
- ☐ Neck Aches

Mood:

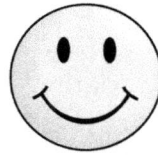

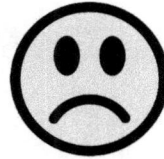

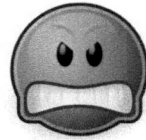

	Things I Did To Feel Better
Day 1	
Day 2	
Day 3	
Day 4	
Day 5	
Day 6	
Day 7	

Notes:

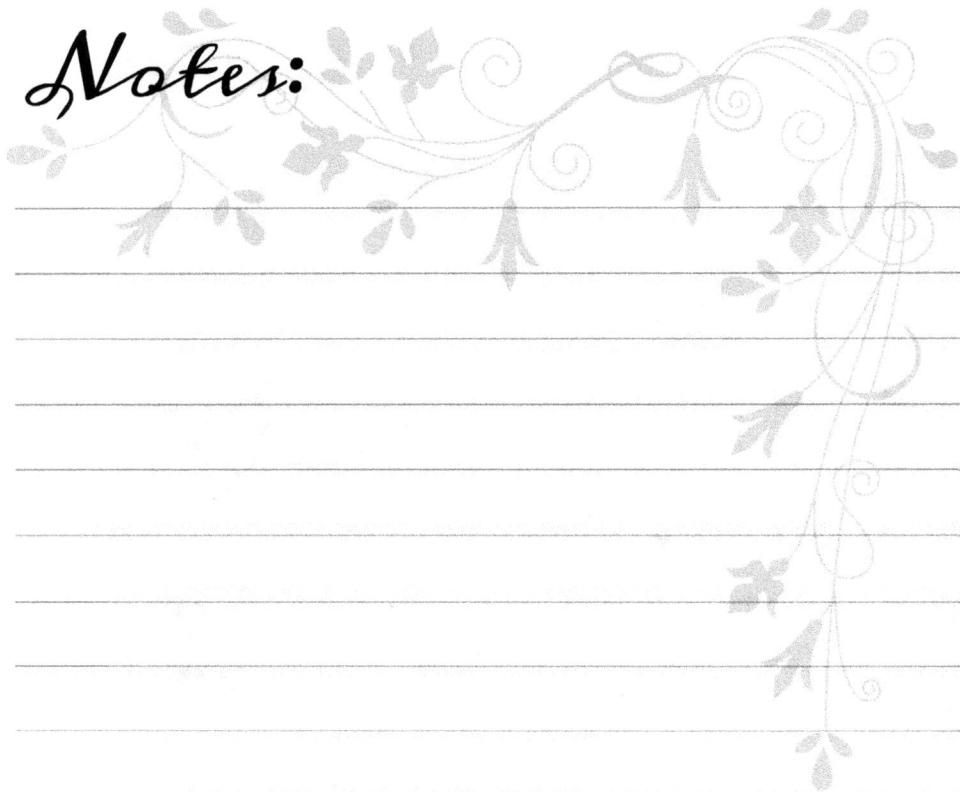

Month:

Year:

Sunday	Monday	Tuesday	Wednesday	Thursday	Friday	Saturday

Days Since Last Period:

Count the number of days in between the 1st day of each cycle. Take the average of several cycles and find out how long your cycles are.

Weight:

Temp:

Symptoms:

- ❏ Cramps
- ❏ Acne
- ❏ Headaches
- ❏ Backaches
- ❏ Bloating
- ❏ Cravings
- ❏ Tender Breasts
- ❏ Nausea
- ❏ Neck Aches

Mood:

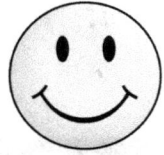

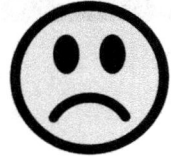

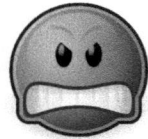

	Things I Did To Feel Better
Day 1	
Day 2	
Day 3	
Day 4	
Day 5	
Day 6	
Day 7	

Notes:

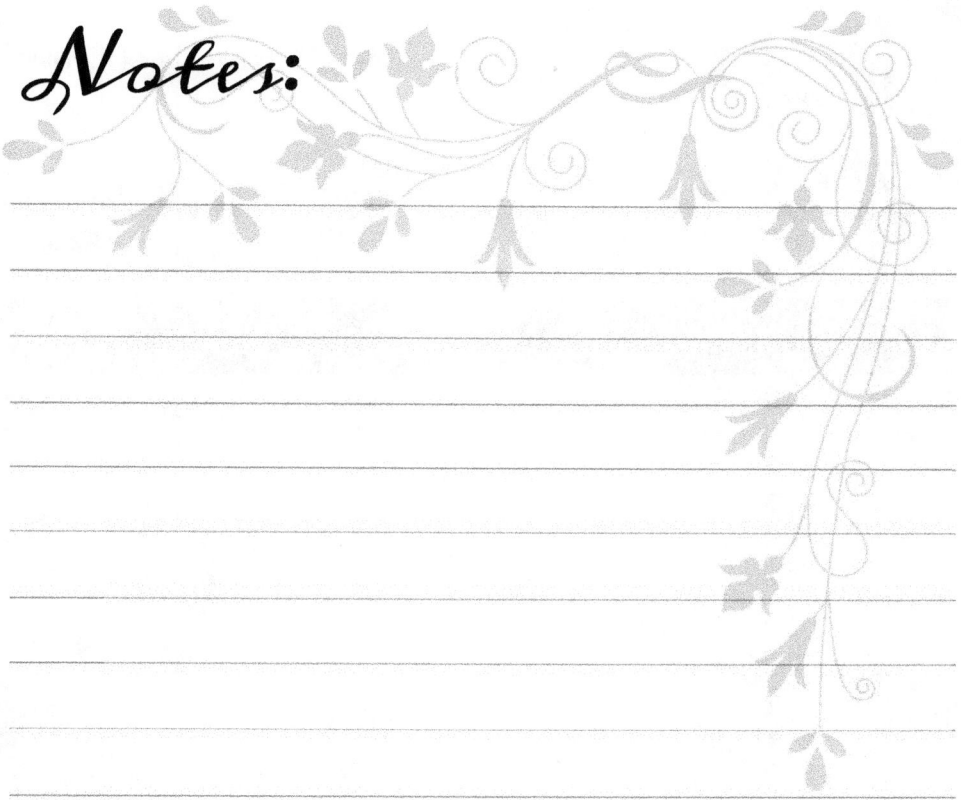

Month:

Year:

Sunday	Monday	Tuesday	Wednesday	Thursday	Friday	Saturday

Days Since Last Period:

Count the number of days in between the 1st day of each cycle. Take the average of several cycles and find out how long your cycles are.

Weight:

Temp:

- ☐ Cramps
- ☐ Acne
- ☐ Headaches
- ☐ Backaches
- ☐ Bloating
- ☐ Cravings
- ☐ Tender Breasts
- ☐ Nausea
- ☐ Neck Aches

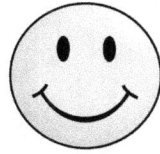

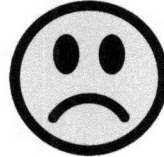

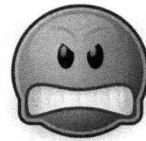

	Things I Did To Feel Better
Day 1	
Day 2	
Day 3	
Day 4	
Day 5	
Day 6	
Day 7	

Notes:

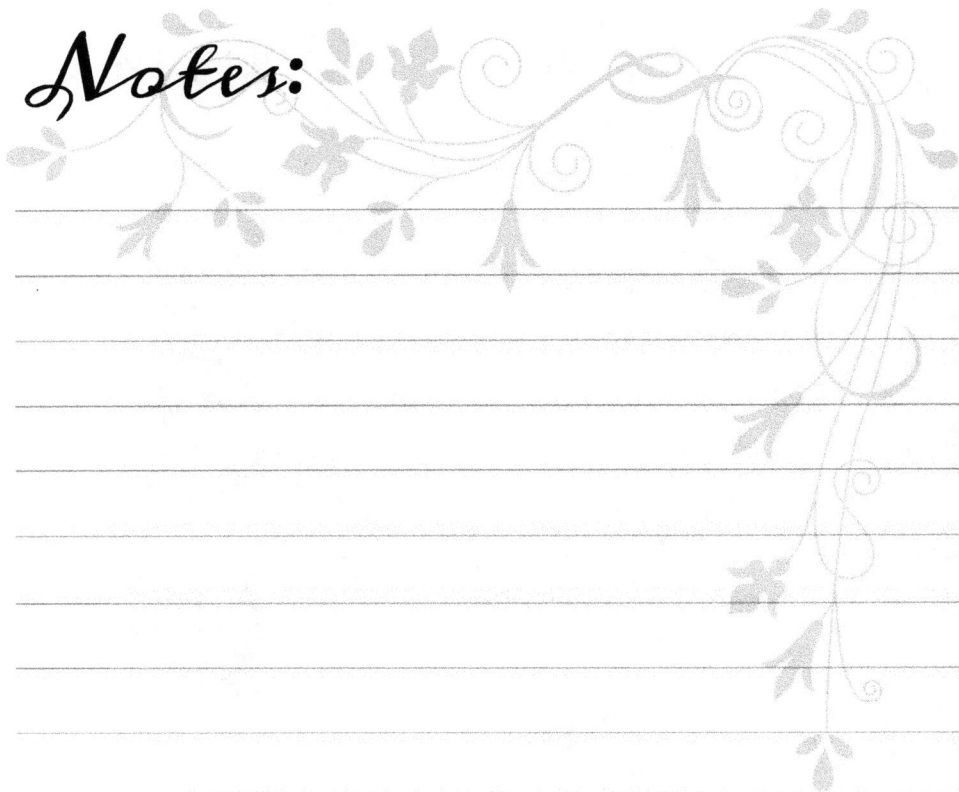

Month:

Year:

Sunday	Monday	Tuesday	Wednesday	Thursday	Friday	Saturday

Days Since Last Period:

Count the number of days in between the 1st day of each cycle. Take the average of several cycles and find out how long your cycles are.

Weight:

Temp:

Symptoms:

- ❏ Cramps
- ❏ Acne
- ❏ Headaches
- ❏ Backaches
- ❏ Bloating
- ❏ Cravings
- ❏ Tender Breasts
- ❏ Nausea
- ❏ Neck Aches

Mood:

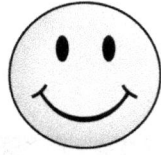

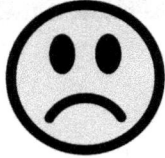

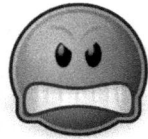

	Things I Did To Feel Better
Day 1	
Day 2	
Day 3	
Day 4	
Day 5	
Day 6	
Day 7	

Notes:

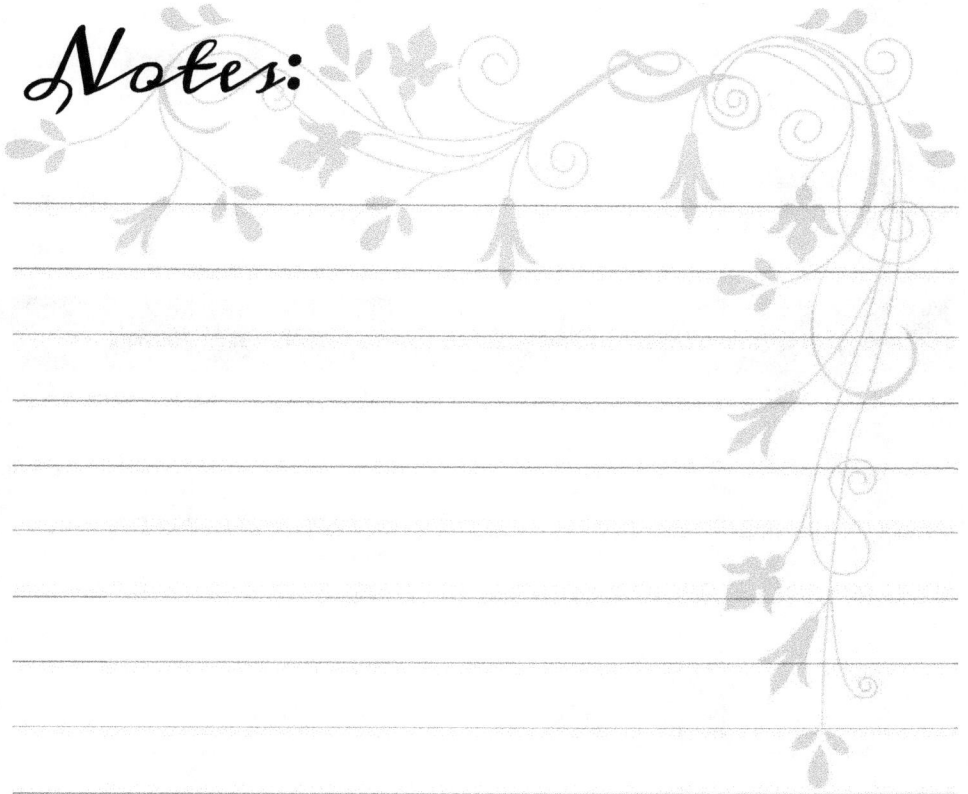

Month:

Year:

Sunday	Monday	Tuesday	Wednesday	Thursday	Friday	Saturday

Days Since Last Period:

Count the number of days in between the 1st day of each cycle. Take the average of several cycles and find out how long your cycles are.

Weight:

Temp:

Symptoms:

- ❏ Cramps
- ❏ Acne
- ❏ Headaches
- ❏ Backaches
- ❏ Bloating
- ❏ Cravings
- ❏ Tender Breasts
- ❏ Nausea
- ❏ Neck Aches

Mood:

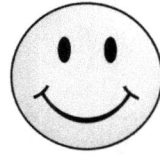

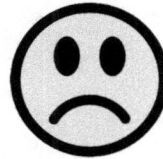

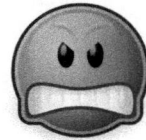

	Things I Did To Feel Better
Day 1	
Day 2	
Day 3	
Day 4	
Day 5	
Day 6	
Day 7	

Notes:

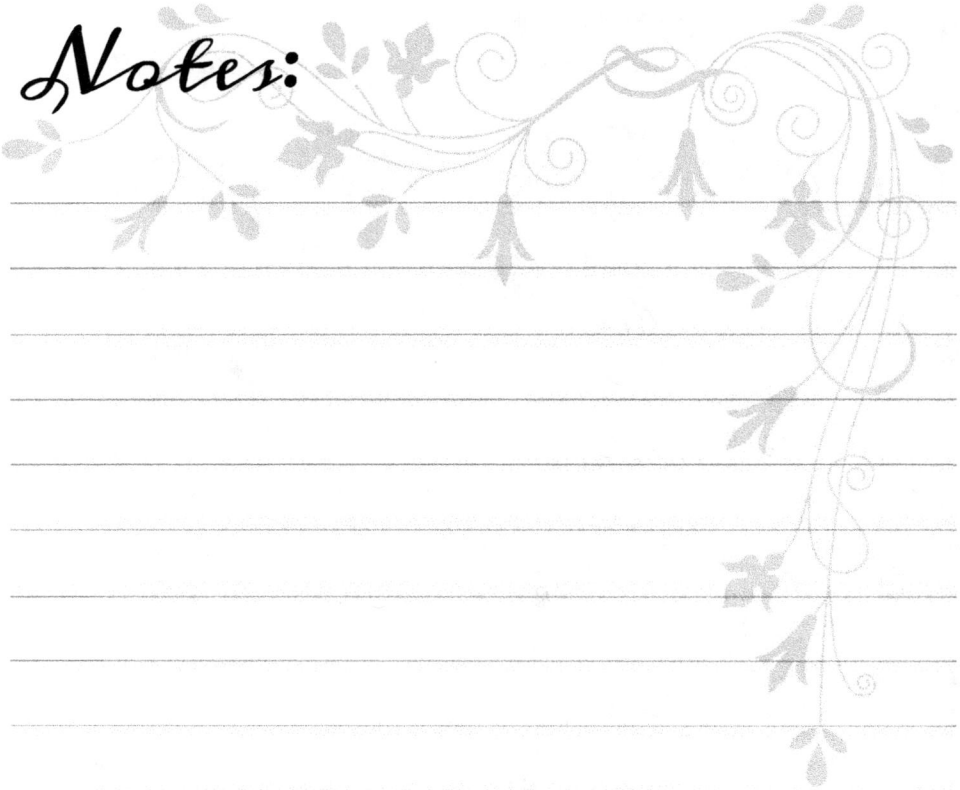

Month:

Year:

Sunday	Monday	Tuesday	Wednesday	Thursday	Friday	Saturday

Days Since Last Period:

Count the number of days in between the 1st day of each cycle. Take the average of several cycles and find out how long your cycles are.

Weight:

Temp:

Symptoms:

- ❏ Cramps
- ❏ Acne
- ❏ Headaches
- ❏ Backaches
- ❏ Bloating
- ❏ Cravings
- ❏ Tender Breasts
- ❏ Nausea
- ❏ Neck Aches

Mood:

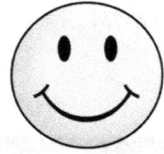

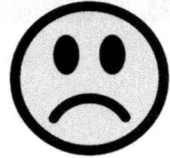

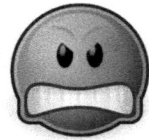

	Things I Did To Feel Better
Day 1	
Day 2	
Day 3	
Day 4	
Day 5	
Day 6	
Day 7	

Notes:

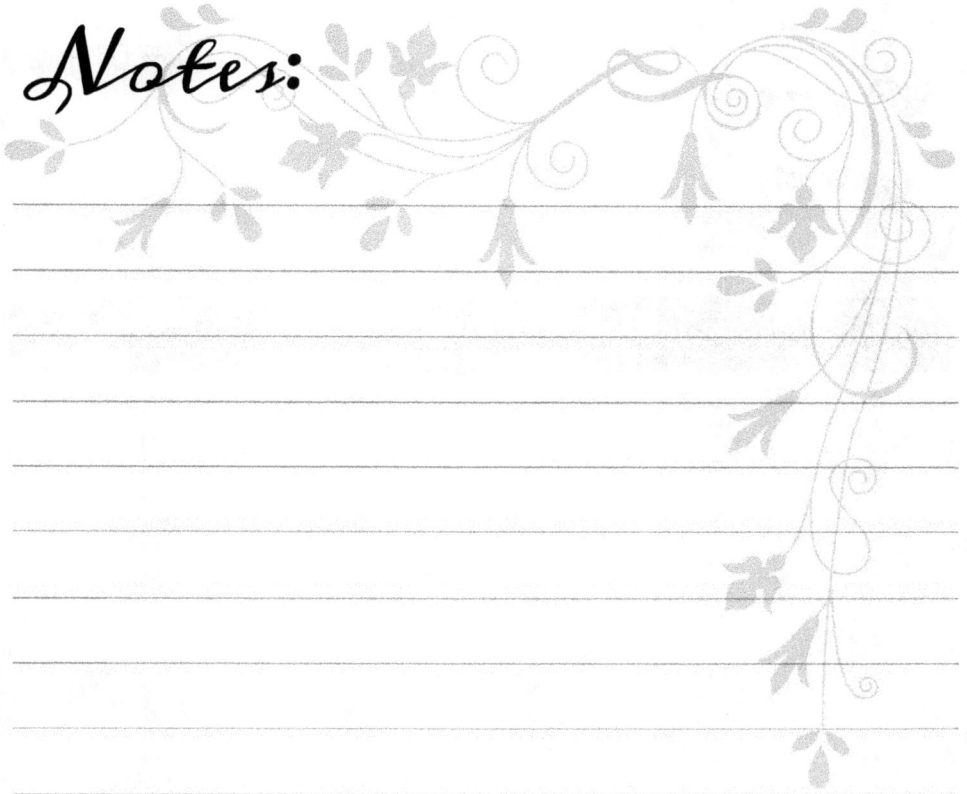

Month:

Year:

Sunday	Monday	Tuesday	Wednesday	Thursday	Friday	Saturday

Days Since Last Period:

Count the number of days in between the 1st day of each cycle. Take the average of several cycles and find out how long your cycles are.

Weight:

Temp:

Symptoms:

- ❏ Cramps
- ❏ Acne
- ❏ Headaches
- ❏ Backaches
- ❏ Bloating
- ❏ Cravings
- ❏ Tender Breasts
- ❏ Nausea
- ❏ Neck Aches

Mood:

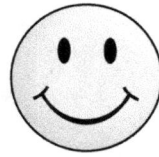

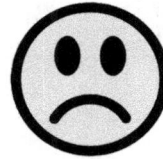

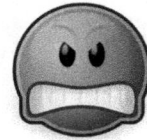

	Things I Did To Feel Better
Day 1	
Day 2	
Day 3	
Day 4	
Day 5	
Day 6	
Day 7	

Notes:

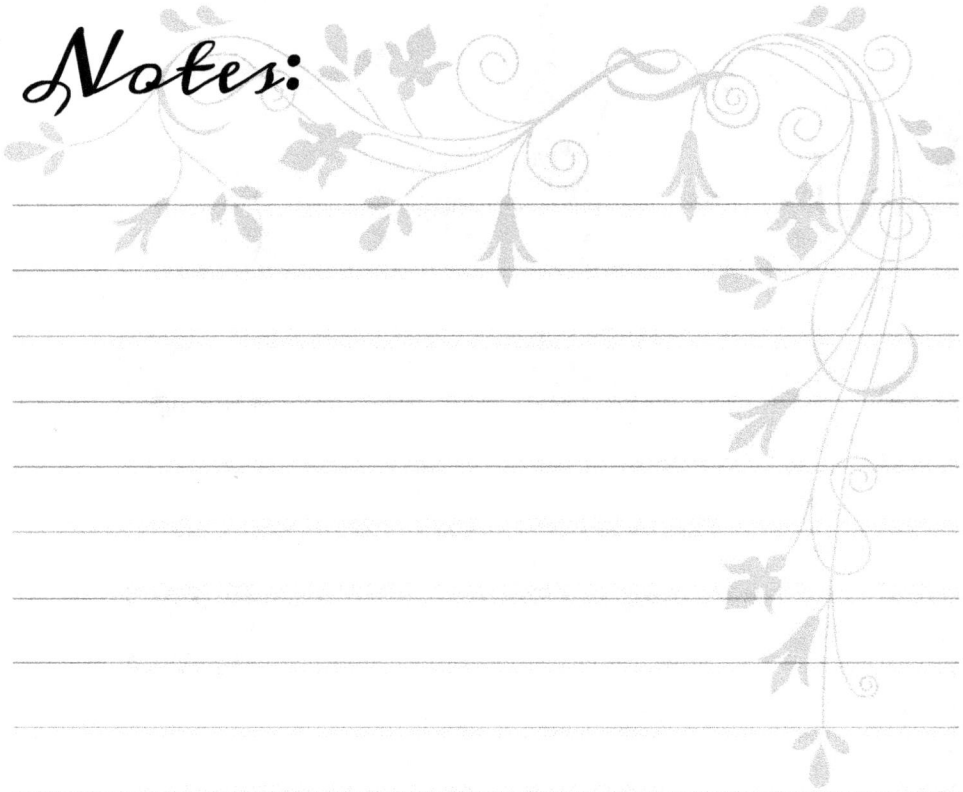

Month:

Year:

Sunday	Monday	Tuesday	Wednesday	Thursday	Friday	Saturday

Days Since Last Period:

Count the number of days in between the 1st day of each cycle. Take the average of several cycles and find out how long your cycles are.

Weight:

Temp:

Symptoms:

- ❏ Cramps
- ❏ Acne
- ❏ Headaches
- ❏ Backaches
- ❏ Bloating
- ❏ Cravings
- ❏ Tender Breasts
- ❏ Nausea
- ❏ Neck Aches

Mood:

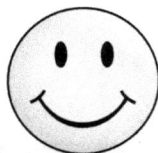

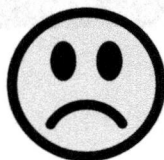

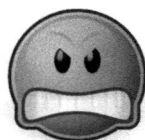

	Things I Did To Feel Better
Day 1	
Day 2	
Day 3	
Day 4	
Day 5	
Day 6	
Day 7	

Notes:

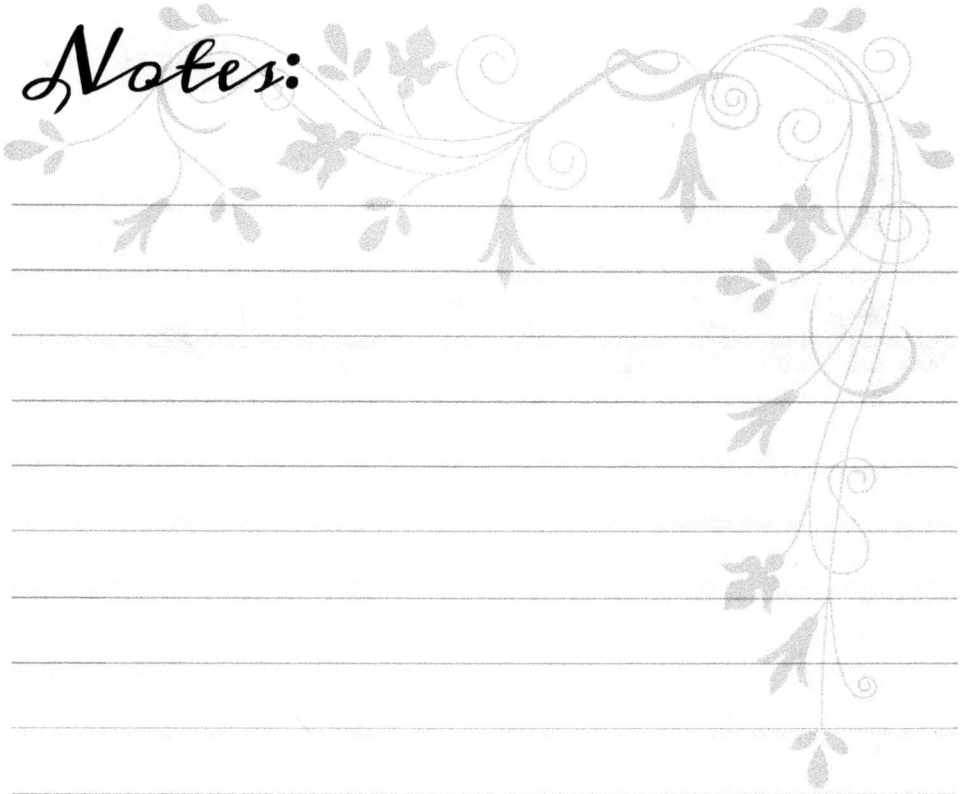

Month:

Year:

Sunday	Monday	Tuesday	Wednesday	Thursday	Friday	Saturday

Days Since Last Period:

Count the number of days in between the 1st day of each cycle. Take the average of several cycles and find out how long your cycles are.

Weight:

Temp:

Symptoms:

- ❑ Cramps
- ❑ Acne
- ❑ Headaches
- ❑ Backaches
- ❑ Bloating
- ❑ Cravings
- ❑ Tender Breasts
- ❑ Nausea
- ❑ Neck Aches

Mood:

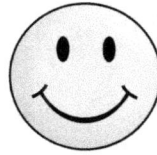

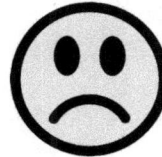

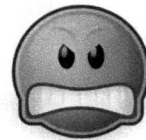

	Things I Did To Feel Better
Day 1	
Day 2	
Day 3	
Day 4	
Day 5	
Day 6	
Day 7	

Notes:

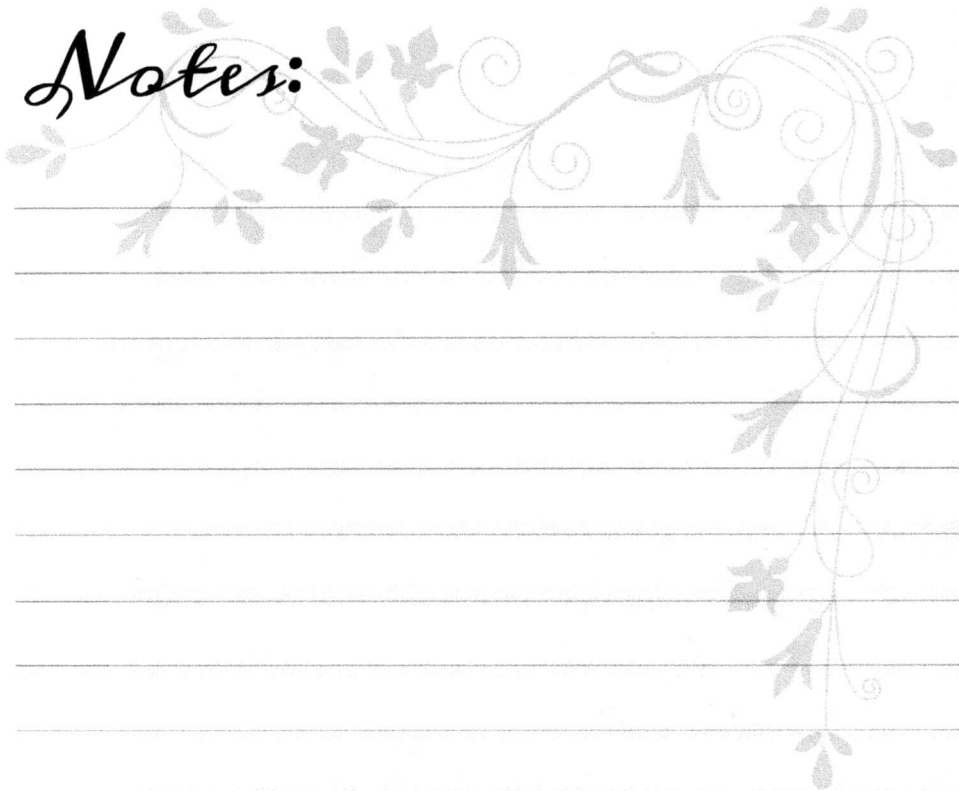

Month:

Year:

Type Of Flow:

L – Light
M – Medium
H – Heavy

Sunday	Monday	Tuesday	Wednesday	Thursday	Friday	Saturday

Days Since Last Period:

Count the number of days in between the 1st day of each cycle. Take the average of several cycles and find out how long your cycles are.

Weight:

Temp:

- ❑ Cramps
- ❑ Acne
- ❑ Headaches
- ❑ Backaches
- ❑ Bloating
- ❑ Cravings
- ❑ Tender Breasts
- ❑ Nausea
- ❑ Neck Aches

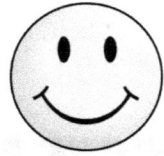

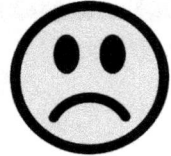

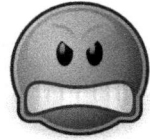

	Things I Did To Feel Better
Day 1	
Day 2	
Day 3	
Day 4	
Day 5	
Day 6	
Day 7	

Notes:

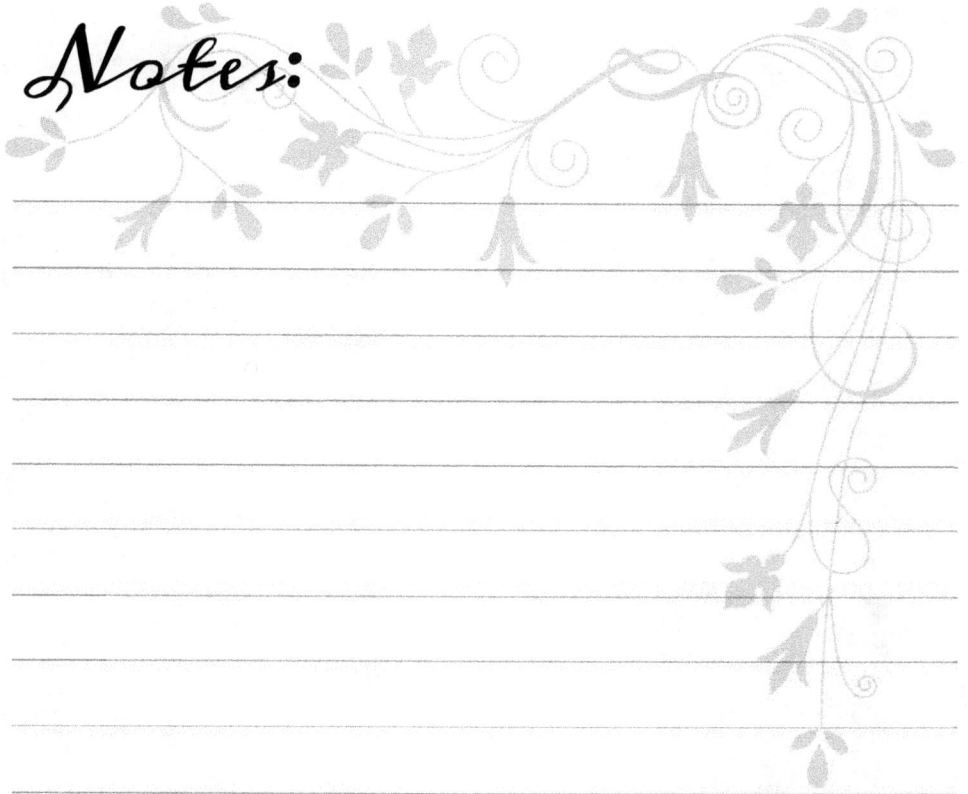

Notes:

www.ingramcontent.com/pod-product-compliance
Lightning Source LLC
Chambersburg PA
CBHW051030030426
42336CB00015B/2809